Dedicated to the underappreciated

M.D. Tophus

Burnout in Healthcare.

Hilphma Publications 2022. www.hilphmapublication.com

First Edition.

Germany.

The author has over 25 years of clinical experience in the healthcare field. Is cognisant of both DSM-5-TR (and previous versions) and ICD-11 (and previous versions) disorders and conditions; quality and safety improvement in healthcare; and healthcare education.

Other M.D. Tophus publications available:

"Exercising Quality in Healthcare Service Provision: A Complex Care Workbook for All Healthcare Professionals." Hilphma Publications: 2022.

"Who is This Colleague?: Dangers of the Healthcare Profession, and beyond. An Interview Guide for Recruitment, Performance Appraisal and Post-Adverse Events." Hilphma Publications: 2022.

"Think on your Feet: Those Who Can. For the Consummate Healthcare Professional." Hilphma Publications: 2022.

"The Unfortunate Healthcare Treater, The Hapless Healthcare Therapist: Narcissistic and Borderline Personality Disorder clients. The Grit." Hilphma Publications: 2022.

"Victims of Crime: Introduction to Forensic Challenges in Healthcare." Hilphma Publications: 2022.

"The A to Z of Workplace Bullying: For the Healthcare Professional and Beyond." Hilphma Publications: 2022.

"Trauma United, Life Defined. A Healthcare Tool for Professionals Across the Globe." Hilphma Publications: 2022.

"Reflective Thinking: the True Healthcare Tool." Hilphma Publications: 2022.

CONTENTS

Page

INTRODUCTION

Burnout is a syndrome which is not embraced in the healthcare field- lest it promotes the perception that one is- weak, incapable, unprofessional, mad, or has chosen the wrong profession.

These perceptions could not be further from the truth. The extensive professional and personal qualities of the burntout healthcare professional have, and continue to be present, but when one is suffering from burnout they can appear well hidden, and feel inaccessable to the sufferer.

The consequences of emotional and physical exhaustion overshadow the healthcare professional's capacity for healthy occupational functioning, creating a haze which feels impenetrable and irreparable.

Overflow, professional exhaustion and overstraining, are just some of the other terms used to connote the state of burnout in for instance, workforces.

Heavy workloads, low autonomy, minimal collegial support, lengthy work hours and overtime, poor management/leadership, limited resources and negative working environments (such as bullying)- at the least- can create enduring fatigue, high stress, insomnia, significant physiological issues, depression, apathy and much more in the healthcare worker. This in turn, effects work functioning: productivity, safety and quality of work undertaken, and realisation of ethical healthcare to the point of lengthy absenteeism, inability to attend to work tasks, feelings of failure, and high levels of cynicism toward healthcare.

In many countries, workers' mental health and well-being (and the conceptualisation of burnout) has been acknowledged via occupational safety and health type discussions along with work stress and burnout prevention programmes, whether it is federally, localised or professional body initiated.

This publication covers burnout: symptoms; warning signs; repercussions; assessment; leadership and occupational departments; recovery; preventative measures; healthcare systems; weaponisation of; and, differential diagnoses. It also includes test questions incorporating the key factors explored throughout this book.

Burnout symptoms

Burnout is included in the ICD-11 as an 'occupational phenomenon' (1). Please note, that the syndrome, which is considered a result of unsuccessfully managed chronic workplace stress, is not classified as a medical condition.

"It is characterized by three dimensions:

feelings of energy depletion and exhaustion;

increased mental distance from one's job, or feelings of negativism or cynicism related to one's job; and

reduced professional efficacy" (1).

The syndrome is not applicable to other areas of life functioning. It is work focussed, only.

Issues contributing to burnout: are human factors related. For instance, workplace milieu, style and effectiveness of leadership, capacity of resources, teamwork, expectations of efficiency levels within the workplace, and workflow processes.

Symptoms are in the realms of depersonalization, emotional exhaustion and feelings of decreased personal accomplishment in work activities.

Though not considered a medical condition (it depends upon the country- multiple consider it an occupational disease), it can be argued that many of the individual symptoms (and physical and emotional impacts) of burnout, can fall into different medical condition categories.

For instance, "hypercholesterolemia, type 2 diabetes, coronary heart disease,... cardiovascular disorder, musculoskeletal pain,....pain experiences, prolonged fatigue, headaches, gastrointestinal issues, respiratory problems and mortality below the age of 45 years" (2).

This is in addition to sleep disorders, and depression, following chronic stress. There are higher risks of: injury; obesity; and, increased alcohol use.

Some of the following symptoms are interrelated between categories:

Cynicism- Depersonalization symptoms:

-emotionally or physically numbed

-negative attitude toward patients, healthcare systems

-feeling in 'another world' or seperate from the world, including sensorily

-sensory overload or hyperalert to one's surroundings, or vice versa

-cynical attitudes and behaviors

-impersonal with patients

-high negativity

-distortions in length of time

-distortions in length of distance.

Emotional exhaustion symptoms:

-insomnia

-minimal to no motivation

-lack of energy

-extreme fatigue

-forgetfulness

-poor concentration

-anxiety

-depression

-irritability, anger

-low levels of hopefulness

-sense of dread

-appetite changes

-dream like state

-suicidal ideation.

Issues with professional efficacy- Feelings of decreased personal accomplishment in work activities symptoms:

-tension during completion of basic and complex tasks

-constant feelings of failure

-disinterest (for eg in patients)

-unable to deal with problems

-overwhelmed

-hypercritical of self

-feeling that are frequently making errors, contrary to feedback

-unhelpful, concrete thinking (for instance, to cure or fail)

-negative self-assessment

-low confidence

-inability to persist/ persevere

-low resiliency.

Three different subtypes of burnout have been proposed:
"the exhausted subtype, the exhausted/cynical subtype, and the burned-out subtype, which might represent patients at different developmental stages in the burnout cycle" (3).

Recognise the warning signs of burnout

Shaking

Stressed and worried all the time

Increasing sadness

Unable to sleep, or hypersomnia

Exhaustion, low energy

Increasingly deadened emotions

Persistently tired

Drained: emotionally and physically

Absent minded

Work tasks delayed

Mood swings

Resentful about work

More frequent physical illness, or symptoms (for instance, cold, influenza, headaches, heart palpitations)

Intensifying emotional responses to small issues

After rest, feel that have not recovered

Obsessive-compulsive, or increased perfectionistic, tendencies

Burnout repercussions

Work:

-poor quality of care;

-medical errors;

-reduced job dissatisfaction.

Personal life:

-affects on all areas of life functioning in addition to occupational:
social and familial.

Life functioning, development of:

-emotional dysregulation;

-depressive disorders;

-anxiety disorders; and/or

-long-term fatigue;

The Burnout Measure- short version (BMS-10)

-10 items

Assesses:

    -physical, mental, emotional exhaustion;

    -hopelessness;

    -appetite;

    -work enthusiasm;

    -sleep;

    -control

(8).

The Burnout Screening Scales (BOSS)

-3 subscales

-Scales I and II: 30 items

Scale I:

    -work impact;

    -personal, family, friends;

    -psychological, physical and psycho-social symptoms

Scale II: bodily, cognitive and emotional symptoms

(9).

The Bergen Burnout Indicator-15 (BBI-15) short measure

-15 items

Measures:

-work based exhaustion;

-cynicism;

-feelings of inadequacy

-specific to occupational health

(10).

Burnout Dimensions Inventory (BODI)

-has 4 domains

Measures:

-resilience, resistance and overload;

-dissociation;

-boundaries;

-depression;

-dysfunctional compensation

(11).

Shirom-Melamed Burnout Measure (SMBM)

Assesses:

  -exhaustion;

  -burnout;

  -health risks

-14 items

Items include:

  -physical fatigue;

  -emotional exhaustion;

  -cognitive weariness/ tiredness

(12).

Workplace/Occupational absenteeism/ Off-work assessment

This is highly dependant upon state and country laws along with occupational/ professional body guidelines.

Potentially: BAT or MBI.

Further Test examples for Depersonalization:

-Beck Depression Inventory-II (BDI-II)

It measures the:

-physiological;

-cognitive;

-affective;

-motivation

elements of depression (13).

Further Test example for emotional exhaustion:

-The Karolinska Exhaustion Disorder Scale (KEDS)

-9 items

Measures:

  -concentration;

  -memory;

  -physical stamina;

-mental stamina;

-recovery;

-sleep;

-hypersensitivity sensorily;

-experience of demands;

-irritation;

-anger.

Assessment specific for exhaustion in clinical (and research environments)
(14).

Further Test example encompassing reduced accomplishment or professional efficacy:

-Burnout Assessment Tool (BAT).

Warning signs/ pre-burnout testing:

-Coping scales;

-occupational stress assessments;

-workplace satisfaction scales;

-workplace anxiety measures

-occupational stress scales;

-depression assessments.

Burnout and leadership, human resources/ occupational departments

Burnout is considered such a vast problem that the World Health Organization (1) has acknowledged it within the realms of a significant and serious phenomenon.

Paperwork

Some alternative descriptions of burnout, dependent upon state and country, are:

-negligent infliction of emotional occupational distress;

-workplace fatigue and distress; physical and mental trauma;

-mental stress, mental strain.

Supplemental information, includes:

-bullying and harrassment claims;

-medical diagnosis of depression resultant from occupational stress;

-demonstrative lack of managerial support, for example in: organisational
 change, role change, workload, working patterns; occupational/burnout syndrome leading
 to psychological injuries.

In relation to workplace claims (again, depending very much upon the jurisdiction), the following may be helpful:

-evidentiary photographs;

-witness statements;

-medical reports;

-special damages claims' documentation;

-legal representation.

Upon workplace injury:

-speaking with one's doctor

-discussion with employer (seek legal advice, perhaps, before speaking to employer)

-time off, need for psychological assessment to prove claim/if considering lengthy sick leave,

are examples of the process.

Understanding the symptoms and impact on work functioning (and capacity for longevity when unable to take time off from work), are necessary.

Risk factors

-continued excessive workload

-decreased autonomy and control over workload

-unreasonable demands

-lengthy, poorly compensated work hours

-minimal breaks along with the individual physical, psychological and emotional symptoms increasing toward burnout.

Work duties, team work- leadership

-transformational leadership is best to reduce chances of burnout, especially in high pressure work environments (it involves individual attention/ consideration for the worker, and intellectual stimulation)

-transactional, servant or passive, leadership are generally not helpful to minimise high burnout rates.

Recovering from burnout

Time off

Mental well-being activities

Adjusting coping resources

Preventative measures to reduce risk of future burnout

Clear boundaries between work and personal life

Possibility of flexible work hours

Testing for recovery from burnout example: Recovery Stress Questionnaire for Work (RESTQ-Work)

-can be utilised when rehabilitating/recovering from work stress/burnout

-the RESTQ Work 55:

- has 55 items

-measures threat resistant stress/strain, and resources

7 different domains encompassing:

-socio-emotional stress;

-performance stress;

-overall recovery;

-burnout/loss of meaning;

-breaks;

-psychosocial recovery;

-work based recovery

(15).

Burnout and healthcare systems

Team impact

-increased and frequent conflict

-inadvertent modelling of high stress

-high stress becomes the 'norm'

-increased levels of negative reactivity in response to extreme workplace demands.

Leadership and management impact

-task dissemination difficulties

-impact on leaders/managers if have poor work productivity within team/s

-tasks delay

-significant and prolonged inefficiencies.

Healthcare facility impact

-bottom-up effects from affected employees to leaders/managers to team to (for instance) wards to healthcare units to healthcare facility/ies.

Economic impact

-healthcare costs

-patient safety and quality, and compromisation of healthcare ethical standards can lead to higher mortality and morbidity rates and thus, litigation, and nil re-accreditation.

Work retention rates impact

-staff retention problems

-high staff turnover

-lengthy absenteeism

-job role changes.

Reputational impact on healthcare facility/system

-difficulty recruiting new healthcare workers

-reduced patient referrals

-reduced healthcare funding

-external healthcare facility/ies' audits

-patient avoidance.

Misdiagnoses, differential diagnoses of Burnout

Diagnoses post-onset of Burnout

Differential diagnosis: adjustment disorder, mood disorders or, anxiety, related disorders.

This incorporates both ICD-11 and DSM-5-TR (17) disorders. Please note, the following are mere examples of some of the assessable disorders related to (or as alternatives) to the diagnosis of burnout/burnout syndrome; and a targetted summary, only.

Adjustment disorder

ICD-11:

      -identifiable psycho-social stressor/s with:

      excessive worry;

      failure to adapt;

      rumination regarding current stressors; and,

      significant impairment in occupational and/or other areas of life functioning.

      -symptoms occur within 1 month of the stressor

(1).

DSM-5-TR:

-emotional or behavioral symptoms in response to a stressor/s which are:
disproportionate to the severity of distress; or,
significant impairment in occupational, social or other areas of life functioning.

-is differentiated from bereavement.

-onset of symptoms are within 3 months of the stressor/s
(17).

Mood disorders:

ICD-11:

Single episode depressive disorder

-nil history of depressive episodes

-depressed mood, or
diminished interest in activities
hopelessness
fatigue
appetite changes
alterations in sleep patterns.

Mixed depressive and anxiety disorder

       -depression

       -anxiety

       -significant distress, or
        impairment in areas of life functioning, eg occupational

(1).

DSM-5-TR:

Major depressive disorder with atypical features

       -depression

       -irregular sleep patterns, or
        hypersomnia
        weight gain
        mood can lift with occurrence of positive events

(17).

Anxiety disorders

ICD-11:

Panic disorder

-recurrent panic attacks with the following symptom/s:
heart palpitations/increased heart rate
shortness of breath
shaking
dizziness
sense of doom.

-intense fear
fear of recurrence of panic attacks.

Generalised Anxiety Disorder

-excessive worry focussed on:
multiple daily events

-anxiety symptoms.

Specific Phobia

-marked excessive fear or anxiety
upon exposure to situations or objects.

-example of objects: sight of blood or injury.

Also,Secondary mood syndromes.
(1).

DSM-5-TR:

Panic disorder

-avoidance of social situations, including work

-withdrawal from situations for fear of having a panic attack, and the
reactions from others to the panic attack

-in addition to the above physiological symptoms, derealization (feelings
of unreality) or depersonalization (a sense of detachment)

-1 or more attacks, with at least one month of intense fear of
recurrence.

Generalized anxiety disorder

-excessive anxiety and worry

-fatigue
irritability
gastrointestinal issues
sleep difficulties

-can overlap with depressive symptomatology.

Specific phobia

-extreme or irrational fear/s, avoidance and anxiety

-specific stimulus based

-negatively impacts normal routine, including if the stimulus is within the work environment (for instance, medical procedures)

-anxiety based symptoms

-2 relevant categories: situational, or other, specific phobias

(17).

ABBREVIATIONS

ASD: Acute Stress Disorder

AWS: Areas of Worklife Survey

BAT: Burnout Assessment Tool

BAT-C: Burnout Assessment Tool- Core Dimensions

BAT-S: Burnout Assessment Tool- Secondary Dimensions

BBI: Bergen Burnout Indicator

BDI-II: Beck Depression Inventory-II

BMS-10: Burnout Measure Short version 10

BODI: Burnout Dimensions Inventory

BOSS: Burnout Screening Scales

CPTSD: Complex Post-Traumatic Stress Disorder

DSM-5- TR: Diagnostic and Statistical Manual for Mental Disorders- 5 Text Revision

ICD-11: International Statistical Classification of Diseases and Related Health Problems-11

KEDS: Karolinska Exhaustion Disorder Scale

MBI-HSS (MP): Maslach Burnout Inventory Human Services Survey for Medical Personnel

MBI-HSS: Maslach Burnout Inventory Human Services Survey

OLBI: Oldenburg Burnout Inventory

PTSD: Post-Traumatic Stress Disorder

REST Q Work 55: Recovery Stress Questionnaire for Work 55

SMBM: Shirom-Melamed Burnout Measure

SVS: Second Victim Syndrome

INDEX

REFERENCES

(1) World Health Organization (2019), International Statistical Classification of Diseases and Related Health Problems, 11th ed,; ICD-11.

(2) Salvagioni, A.D.J., Melanda, F.N., Mesas, A.E., Gonzalez, A.D., Gabani, F.L. and Andrade, S.M.d. (2017). Physical, psychological and occupational consequences of job burnout: A systematic review of prospective studies. PLoS ONE 12 (10) e0185781: 1-29.

(3) Bauernhofer, K., Bassa, D., Canazei, M., Jimenez, P., Paechter, M., Papousek, I., Fink, A. and Weiss, E.M. (2018). Subtypes in clinical burnout patients enrolled in an employee rehabilitation program: difference in burnout profiles, depression, and recovery/resources-stress balance. BMC Psychiatry, 18, 10.

(4) Maslach, C., Jackson, S.E., Leiter, P., Schaufeli, W.B. and Schwab, R.L. (2022). Maslach Burnout Inventory (MBI). www.mindgarden.com

(5) Kristensen, T.S., Borritz, M., Villadsen, E. and Christensen, K.B. (2005). The Copenhagen Burnout Inventory: A new tool for the assessment of burnout. Work and Stress, 19: 192-207.

(6) Schaufeli, W.B., Desart, S. and De Witte, H. (2020). Burnout Assessment Tool (BAT)- Development, validity and reliability. International Journal of Environmental Research and Public Health, 17, 9495: 1-21.

(7) Demorouti, E. and Bakker, A.B. (2008). The Oldenburg Burnout Inventory: A good alternative to measure burnout and engagement. In Handbook of Stress and Burnout in Healthcare, pp.65-78. www.psicopolos.com/burnout/bumesur.pdf

(8) Malach-Pines, A. (2005). The Burnout Measure, short version. International Journal of Stress Management, 12(1): 78-88.

(9) Geuerich, K. and Hagemann, W. (2014). Burnout Screening Scale I, II and III. www.testzentrale.de

(10) Näätänen, P., Aro, A., Matthiesen, S. and Salmela-Aro, K. (2003). Bergen Burnout Indicator 15. Edita, Helsinki.

(11) Scheibenbogen, O., Andorfer, U., Kuderer, M. and Musalek, M. (2017). Prävelenz des Burnout-Syndroms in Österreich. Verlaufsformen und relevante Präventions-und Behandlungs- strategien. Bundesministerium für Arbeit, Soziales, Gesundheit und Konsumentenschutz, Vienna.

(12) Shirom, A. and Melamed, S. (2006). A comparison of the construct validity of two burnout measures in two groups of professionals. International Journal of Stress Management, 13(2): 176-200.

(13) Beck, A.T., Steer, R.A. and Brown, G.K. (1996). BDI-II: Beck depression inventory manual. 2nd edn. San Antonio, TX: Psychological Corporation.

(14) Beser, A., Sorjonen, K., Walhberg, K., Peterson, U., Nygren, A. and Asberg, M. (2014). Construction and evaluation of a self rating scale for stress-induced Exhaustion Disorder, the Karolinska Exhaustion Disorder Scale. Scand. J. Psychol. Feb, 55(1): 72-82.

(15) Jimenez, P. and Kallus, K.W. (2016). Recovery-Stress Questionnaire for Work (RESTQ- Work). Frankfurt am Main: Pearson Assessent and Information GmbH.

(16) Tophus, M.D. (2022). The A to Z of Workplace Bullying: For the Healthcare Professional and Beyond. Hilphma Publications.

(17) American Psychiatric Association (2022), Diagnostic and Statistical Manual of Mental Disorders, 5th ed Text Revision: DSM-5-TR. Washington, D.C.: American Psychiatric Association Publishing.

(18) Tophus, M.D. (2022). Trauma United, Life Defined. A Healthcare Tool for Professionals Across the Globe. Hilphma Publications.

Printed in Great Britain
by Amazon

40811377R00046